Spanish Influenza

(PAN-ASTHENIA)

ITS CAUSE and CURE

By Dr. Louis Dechmann

Author of: Procreation (*Within the Bud*)
Regeneration (*Dare to be Healthy*)
Valere Aude (*Compendium of Dare to be Healthy*)

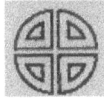

"I attempt a difficult work, but there is no
excellence without difficulty."—*Ovid*

Copyrighted 1919

By THE WASHINGTON PRINTING CO.
Seattle, Washington

Dedication

TO MY GUIDING STARS:

Hippocrates, Boerhaave, Johannes Mueller, Von Liebig and Hensel, I gladly dedicate this work. Thus I attempt to repay in part the debt which humanity owes to these sons of all the ages.

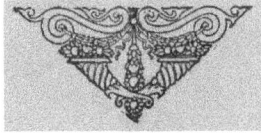

Contents

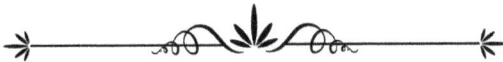

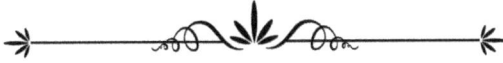

I.

THE REASON FOR MEDICAL FAILURE IN COPING WITH SPANISH INFLUENZA

The Spanish influenza pandemia which is encircling the globe and claiming the lives of hundreds of thousands, aye, of millions of people, presents a problem before which the medical profession stands baffled. A multitude of hypotheses have been offered as a basis for as many methods of treating the plague, but the disease runs its course unchecked. Thus far the medical faculty of the world has not even succeeded in defining the nature of the disease. The first problem, therefore, at least the first aspect of the problem, is to ascertain the nature of the disease, to uncover its underlying cause, in order that we may have a scientific foundation on which to base our diagnosis and our treatment of it.

The purpose of this treatise, therefore, must be two-fold, namely to lay bare the underlying cause of Spanish influenza, and to offer a therapeutic method calculated to remove that cause. The primary phase of our purpose could be stated dogmatically in very few words, but that would leave room for doubt as to the soundness of the premises of our argument, and to remove all possibility of doubt it will be necessary to discuss certain aspects of anatomy and physiology as well as pathology and therapy.

The longest road is sometimes the shortest way to the goal!

Only a few days ago, to-wit, on January 20th, The Seattle Post-Intelligencer published a two column report from the pen of Frederick J. Haskin, Washington, D.

C., detailing the complete failure of a series of experiments made under direction of the Public Health Service Department of the United States Government. He stated that the failure of one hundred men to take the disease during the course of experiments which involved even smearing their throats and noses with matter taken from the throats of patients suffering from the disease had completely baffled the physicians in charge. The widespread publicity given to this report cannot fail to shake the confidence of the general public in the medical profession somewhat.

We know that there is sharp criticism of the profession by the laity, which finds expression in unexpected places. George Bernard Shaw, the distinguished English writer, in a closely reasoned article on the subject of the medical fetish and failure in stolidly complacent England, says : "The assumption is that the 'registered doctor' or surgeon knows everything that is known, and can do everything that is done. This means that the dogma of omniscience, omnipotence, and infallibility, and something very like the theory of apostolic succession and kingship by anointment, have recovered in medicine the grip they have lost in theology and politics. This would not matter if the 'legally qualified doctor' was a *completely qualified healer;* but this is not the case ; far from it. Dissatisfaction with the orthodox methods and technique is so widespread that the supply of technically qualified unregistered practitioners is insufficient for the demand—and some of them draw fees ten to twenty times as large as the registered practitioners. The reputation of the unregistered specialist is usually well-founded. *He must deliver the goods.* He cannot live by the faith of his patients, in a string of letters after his name........"

This is severe criticism in which G. B. S. indulges, but in view of the growth of new schools of healing, and in view of the birth of a new freak of health reform almost every day, there can be little doubt, I take it, that there is a measure of truth in his strictures. There is no need of cataloging either the heterodox schools of healing or the latest additions to the list of freak health reforms, as every physician and most well informed laymen are well acquainted with them. The very fact that the practitioners of these heterodox schools find patients, and the fact that the originators of these freak health reforms find followers, offers ample evidence of loss of faith in orthodox medical practice !

What must be done to curb this tendency ? How shall the shaken confidence of the general public in the medical profession be restored? Whatever is to be done, must be done immediately! It is my hearty desire to assist in restoring confidence. But an enduring faith, confidence, must be justified by works!

In these circumstances I shall speak as frankly and plainly as the facts seem to justify, and all I ask is that my words shall be weighed in the light of my purpose.

This may appear to be a digression from the subject in hand, but it is essential that we take a bird's eye view of the whole field before we confine ourselves to consideration of the particular problem which is our theme.

There is, of course, a fundamental difference between the viewpoint of this treatise and that of the medical fraternity in general in examining the problem presented by the pandemia of Spanish influenza. I can only ask, in advance, that the physician whose point of view differs from mine will suspend judgment until he has read and weighed well the whole of my argument.

/8

It seems to me that there is too much antique mystery in connection with the practice of modern medicine, and too free use of a multitude of drugs which are expected to act as specifics, while all too little attention is paid by the average practitioner to the fundamental problems involved in supplying the nutritive wants of the various tissues of the human body. But on these points I shall let the facts cited in the course of the discussion speak for themselves. I am convinced, however, that the reign of mystery must be ended, and the use of drugs very, very greatly curtailed.

In a report made public on January 12th, the health and morals commissions of Chicago stated that under their direction 741,825 prescriptions written by doctors in October at the height of the influenza epidemic had been examined. Of these prescriptions 441,641 were evidently intended for influenza and pneumonia patients and 104,010 of them contained opium or its derivatives. The report adds that these drugs were unnecessary and dangerous. This is indeed a conservative statement of the case!

An editorial warning against too much confidence in vaccination as a means of combatting Spanish influenza, which appeared in the Journal of the American Medical Association on November 9, 1918, contained the following statements: "Nothing can be learned as to its real value from indiscriminate vaccination of the public. * * * * * Pending developments, nothing should be done by the medical profession that may arouse unwarranted hope among the public and be followed by disappointment and distrust of medical science and the medical profession."

On this same point, permit me to quote the opinion of Dr. Karl F. Meyer, of the Hooper Institute of Medical Research of the University of California, who says: "Serums have not yet been introduced which produce immunity from Spanish influenza. The serums now employed are of no use whatsoever. Even the vaccine formerly employed successfully against pneumonia is not giving satisfactory results in connection with influenza."

"You have no idea" Dr. Meyer adds, "of how really and truly helpless we are. As an example, take the advice given us by public health men when we asked what should be done if the epidemic struck the West. They said 'organize your hospitals and undertakers' and that came true."

In the same statement Dr. Meyer declared that the medical fraternity is in total darkness as to the cause and nature of Spanish influenza, and if proof of the correctness of his utterance is needed it may be found in the declaration of Surgeon General Rupert Blue, of the United States Public Health Service, on December 11th, that "the country need not fear that the influenza epidemic will return ; it has come and gone for good."

These are the statements of experts, the testimony of men who should know whereof they speak. Dr. Karl F. Meyer is an epidemiologist, an expert on epidemics, connected with one of the great university research institutions, but he confesses his ignorance and that of the entire medical fraternity as to the nature of this plague. Granting that Surgeon General Blue's statement may be of some value judged from the standpoint of psycho-therapy, the fact is that the epidemic is still with us, and likely to be with us, though varying in its intensity according as climatological conditions vary, during the next two or three years.

In the November (1918) number of The American Journal of Public Health, Dr. W. A. Evans and Dr. M. O. Heckard, of the Chicago Health Department, call attention to the fact that : "Hirsch's 'Handbook of Historical and Geographical Pathology' records almost one hundred epidemics occurring in the eight hundred years prior to 1889. It is clearly set forth," they declare, "that practically each of these epidemics lasted longer than one year, or else recurred several times during the course of two or more years."

I have not spoken of the use of masks as a preventive measure, but when these much vaunted contraptions are spoken of "it is," as the old proverb says, "very hard not to write a satire." Let us, therefore, try to forget this greatest farce in the entire history of medicine !

There can be no doubt that the medical fraternity knows nothing as to the cause, and very little, if anything, about the nature of Spanish influenza, with the inevitable result that the whole medical world is busy battling against effects. It may be asked, and with very good reason, too, why should medical scientists find themselves in this position? The answer to this pertinent query will be forthcoming presently. Then, we shall resume the trail and attempt to point out the fundamental cause of this plague, and having done that, we shall be in a position to make the nature of the disease clear, and having a clear idea of both its cause and nature, we shall offer a therapeutic plan calculated to remove its cause.

The medical fraternity of the whole world finds itself thrust into a cul de sac by Spanish influenza, thanks to the work of two of the great stars of Germany, namely, Prof. Robert Koch and Prof. Rudolph Virchow! It is not my desire to belittle either the intentions or the labors of these men. On the contrary, I deeply appreciate the sincere motives and the laborious experimental work of both. But so far as the results of their work is concerned, the facts themselves are sufficiently eloquent.

It is thirty years since Prof. Koch, discoverer of the tubercle bacillus, announced that he had found an unfailing cure for tuberculosis, which he named tuberculin. From that day until this hour, medical science has been chasing its bacteriological phantom. But in 1909, before the Tuberculosis Congress at Washington, D. C., Prof. Koch announced that he was still continuing his search for a cure !

As to the value of Prof. Koch's tuberculin, let me quote a single statement from "Medicine" by Dr. Frederick Meyer: "One disease only, alas! the one which costs mankind the heaviest losses, cannot yet, in spite of the most brilliant discoveries of modern times, be presented in a manner at all satisfactory. Tuberculosis has become the worst enemy of our race, innumerable victims of this disease are yearly dissected and examined, and yet it has not hitherto proved possible to determine whether the subjects of tuberculosis are killed by the poisons developed by Koch's bacillus or as a result of infection. * * * * * From these statements it is evident that we have up to the present time no effective serum for use in tuberculosis."

As a matter of fact, Prof. Koch himself has said: "the remedy does not kill the tubercle bacillus, but only the tubercular tissue."

Thirty years ago the German Reichstag gave Prof. Robert Koch a million marks in appreciation of his great discovery of an unfailing cure for the terrible plague, tuberculosis. It did not take thirty years to find the futility of Koch's tuberculin. The immortal Julius Hensel made clear its failure in 1892, just two years after its discovery had been announced with trumpets. In spite of the failure of Prof. Koch to find an unfailing cure in more than thirty years of systematic and laborious work, every student is led to chase the phantom of bacillus and to concoct more serums. It is in order, I think, to ask, why ?

The answer to the foregoing question must lead to consideration of the theory of "Cellular Pathology" formulated by Prof. Robert Virchow, which was published in 1858. This theory, in a nutshell, is that changes in the composition of the cells is the first cause of all disease. He does not give the reason for changes in cell structure. It was this, I may say en passant, which led me to the conclusion that Virchow was not familiar enough with chemistry, especially with organic chemistry, to enable him to give the conditions of disease. The results of this colossal error are with us yet. I shall speak at greater length on this point on another occasion.

Just as I was about to fall into the error of viewing the problem from the same point of view as Virchow, I came upon a lecture by Prof. Schweninger, Privy Councilor to Bismarck, which contained the following statement, and this acted as a guide out of the labyrinth for me :

"In order to understand a sickness or disease and to undertake to thoroughly cure the same," says Professor Schweninger," it is first of all necessary to unfold before one's mental vision the ways and means of its formation, and by degrees to trace its origin, before one is enabled to prepare therapeutic measures conformable to the individual stages of same."

In this sense I strenuously tried to get at the bottom of the inception of constitutional diseases, but the entire medical literature served only to bring me to pathological anatomy, which informs us that the original cause of disease is a change in the form of the cellular elements of various organs, in explanation of which the customary technical terms are used, such as atrophy, degeneration, metamorphosis, etc. But this did not satisfy me ; I reasoned, surely this cannot be the origin of disease.

The cause for the visible changing of tissues must be sought in the conditional interstitial substances which cause the invisible changes or shiftings of the cellular forms, and which are scientifically termed "changed nutritional conditions." This was my course of reasoning : As the cellules, which are the smallest individual elements of the human system, are only products of the blood, and for their composition require different chemical substances in varying quantities, it is obviously necessary to fathom what those chemical elements of the cellules may be, what form they take in their mutual relation to the separate parts of the body, and in what way they enter the organism.

This involves, first of all, a return to the viewpoint of Hippocrates, "the father of Medicine," and a brief examination of the attitude of his three greatest disciples, Galen, Sydenham and Boerhaave towards the problem. This will keep us, as I shall prove, from being sidetracked, from pinning our faith to abstract theories, from falling into the pit of empirical deductions, and hold us to the task of following the phenomena of life from the formation of the blood to the formation of the cells and the various aggregations of cells called organs and tissues. Thus we shall, if it be at all possible, lay bare the underlying causes of pathological phenomena, of disease.

I have already remarked that there is a fundamental difference between the viewpoint of this treatise and that of the medical fraternity in general, but I want to repeat it, and to again ask the physician whose point of view differs from mine to suspend his judgment until he has read and digested my entire argument.

For the purpose of making the difference between my point of view and that of the leaders of the medical faculty clear, it may be well to cite a brief resume of the teachings of Hippocrates, Galen, Sydenham and Boerhaave. The modern medical world acknowledges that the doctrines of these four men is the foundation upon which the practice of healing has been raised to the status of a science, but it is the least essential part of the work of Hippocrates, namely, his statement of theory which has been given prominence, whilst the most important portion of his labors, the practical part, has been neglected and ignored.

The following passages are taken from the article entitled: "History of Medicine" in the Encyclopedia Britannica, 11th Edition, Vol. XVIII, pages 42-51 :

"Hippocrates, called the 'Father of Medicine' lived during the age of Pericles, (495-429 B. C.) and occupied as high a position in medicine as did the great philosophers, orators and tragedians of their respective fields.

"His high conception of the duties and position of the physician and the skill with which he manipulated the materials that were at hand, constituted two important characteristics of Hippocratic medicine. Another was the recognition that disease, as well as health, is a process governed by what we call natural laws, learned by observation, and indicating the direction of recovery. These views of the 'natural history of disease' led to the habit of minute observation and careful interpretation of symptoms, m which the Hippocratic school excelled and has been the model for all succeeding ages, so that even now the true method of clinical medicine may be said to be the method of Hippocrates.

"One of the important doctrines of Hippocrates was the healing power of nature. He did not teach that nature was sufficient to cure disease, but he recognized a natural process of the humours, at least in acute diseases, being first of all *crude* then passing through coction or digestion, and finally being expelled by resolution or crisis through one of the natural channels of the body. The duty of the physician was to 'assist and not to hinder these changes, so that the sick man might conquer the disease with the help of the physician."

"*Galen*, the man from whom the greater part of modern European medicine has flowed, lived about 131 to 201, A. D. He was equipped with all the anatomical, medical and philosophical knowledge of his time; he had studied all kinds of natural curiosities and was in close touch with important political events ; he possessed enormous industry, great practical sagacity, and unbounded literary fluency. At that time there were numerous sects in the medical profession, various dogmatic systems prevailed in medical science, and the social standing of physicians was degraded. He assumed the task of reforming the existing evils and restoring the unity of medicine as it had been understood by Hippocrates, at the same time elevating the dignity of medical practitioners.

"In the explanation and healing of diseases he applied the science of physiology. His theory was based upon the Hippocratic doctrine of humours, but he developed it with marvelous ingenuity. He advocated that the normal condition of the body depended upon a proper proportion of the four elements, hot, cold, wet and dry. The faulty proportions of the same gave rise, not to diseases, but to the occasions for disease. He laid equal stress upon the faulty composition or dysaemia of the blood. He claimed that all diseases were due to a combination of these morbid predis-positions, together with injurious external influences, and thus explained all symptoms and all diseases. He found a name for every phenomenon and a solution for every problem. And though it was precisely in this characteristic that he abandoned scientific methods and practical utility, it was also this quality that gained for him his popularity and prominence in the medical world.

"However, his reputation grew slowly. His opinions were in opposition to those of other physicians of his time. In the succeeding generation he won esteem as a philosopher, and it was only gradually that his system was accepted implicitly. It enjoyed great, though not exclusive predominance until the fall of Roman civilization."

"*Thomas Sydenham,* (1624-1689) was well acquainted with the works of the ancient physicians and had a fair knowledge of chemistry. Whether he had any knowledge of anatomy is not definitely known. He advocated the actual study of disease in an impartial manner, discarding all hypothesis. He repeatedly referred to Hippocrates in his medical methods, and he has quite deservedly been styled the English Hippocrates. He placed great stress on the 'natural history of disease,' just as did his Greek master, and likewise attached great importance to 'epidemic constitution,' that is, the influence of weather and other natural causes on the process of disease. He believed in the healing power of nature to an even greater degree than did Hippocrates. He claimed that disease was nothing more than an effort on the part of nature to restore the health of the patient by the elimination of the morbific matter.

"The reform of practical medicine was affected by men who advocated the rejection of all hypothesis and the impartial study of natural processes, as shown in health and disease. Sydenham showed that these natural processes could be studied and dealt with without being explained, and, by laying stress on facts and disregarding *explanations,* he introduced a method in medicine far more fruitful than any discoveries. Though the dogmatic spirit continued to live for a long time, the reign of standard authority has passed."

"*Boerhaave.* In the latter part of the seventeenth century a physician arose (1668-1738) who was destined to become far more prominent in the medical world than any of the English physicians of the age of Queen Anne, though he differed but little from them in his way of thinking. This was *Hermann Boerhaave.* For many years he was professor of medicine at Leyden, and excelled in influence and reputation not only his greatest forerunners, Montanus of Padua and Sylvius of Leyden, but probably every subsequent teacher. The hospital at Leyden became the centre of medical influence in Europe. Many of the leading English physicians of the 18th century studied there. Boerhaave's method of teaching was transplanted to Vienna through one of his pupils, Gerard Van Swieten, and thus the noted Vienna school of medicine was founded.

"The services of Boerhaave to the progress of medicine can hardly be overestimated. He was the organizer and almost the constructor of the modern method of clinical instruction. He followed the methods of Hipprocrates and Sydenham in his teachings and in his practice. The points of his system that are best known are his doctrines of inflammation, obstruction, and 'plethora.' In the practice of medicine he aimed to make use of all the anatomical and physiological acquisitions of his age, including microscopical anatomy.

"In this respect he differed from Sydenham, for the latter paid but little more attention to modern medicine than to ancient dogma. In some respects he was like Galen, but again different from him, as he did not wish to reduce his knowledge to any definite system. He spent much time in studying the medical classics, though he valued them from an historical standpoint rather than from an authoritative standpoint. It would almost seem that the great task of Boerhaave's life, a combination of ancient and modern medicine, could not be of any real permanent value, and the same might be said of his Aphorisms, in which he gave a summary of the fact that his contributions to the science of medicine form one of the necessary factors in the construction of modern medicine."

I am justified in my course, therefore, by the teachings of these four pillars of the medical world, all of whom dealt with humoral pathology, but were not in the position to enter as deeply into the problem as we are for the simple reason that neither chemistry nor physiology were anywhere nearly as highly developed as they are in our own day.

It was more than a century after the death of Boerhaave that the world was blessed by birth of Johannes Mueller, the son of a poor shoemaker, who became the greatest physiologist the world has produced. His works on the physiology of man were published in 1833-8, and they are the most authoritative and reliable books on this subject. Our scholastic textbooks on this subject are far below Mueller's, both with regard to matter and the manner of presenting it.

The next great light we were blessed with was the anatomist Joseph Hyrtl. Yes, indeed, he was so great that he dared to make the following statement : "For thousands of years medicine has found remedies, but not a single truth, not a single law of life." Vide : Joseph Hyrtl's Textbook of the Anatomy of Man, 1878, page 31, line 30.

Then came the greatest chemist, Justus von Liebig, who gave us the great law of the minimum, that the absence of the tiniest ingredient essential to the growth and functioning of an organ or tissue will result in the degeneration or improper functioning of that organ or tissue.

Shortly before von Liebig laid down his law of the minimum, Professor Jacob Moleschott, noted Dutch physician, declared : "It is one of the chief questions people are always asking of a physician, how to obtain good, healthy and active blood. Put the question as you will, all who occupy their minds with it are brought by experience to acknowledge explicitly, with whatever degree of hesitation and timidity it may occasion, that our powers of thinking, of feeling and of action, and even our very expectation of progeny, are dependent upon our blood, and our blood on proper nutrition."

The next to throw a powerful light upon the problem was Julius Hensel, master of agricultural and physiological chemistry. With pleasure will I quote some of his work presently in connection with my own explanations and leave it to the intelligent reader to pass judgment. Hensel is bound to be acknowledged very soon as immortal ! His greatest work: "Das Leben, seine Grundlage und die Mittel zu seiner Erhaltung," (Life, its Foundation and the Means for its Preservation) has not yet been translated into English to my knowledge. German edition published by Boericke and Tafel, Philadelphia. The first edition was published in Christiania in 1885, the second edition in Philadelphia in 1890. What is it that has prevented the publication of such a monumental work in English in this country? The knowledge this work contains will work a revolution in medical theory and practice once it is generally known. Is it timidity or orthodox fear that has kept Hensel's work in obscurity? Another monumental work of his entitled: "Makrobiotik, oder Unsere Krankheiten und Unsere Heilmittel," (Macrobiotic, or Our Diseases and Our Remedies) was first published in Germany in 1882 ; the second edition in 1892.

Then came Professor Hueppe, of Prague, bacteriologist, who was first assistant to Prof. Robert Koch at the time he discovered the tubercle bacillus. He tried to act as the balance wheel, but the pressure of the medical profession upon Prof. Koch to publish his discovery was too great for Prof. Hueppe's counter efforts. The following statement which he made should have served as a deterrent until positive proof was forthcoming as to the nature of microbes and bacillus. "The cause of disease in the scientific sense is always internal and is what we designate empirically as disposition. The microbes are only the releasing irritants of a specific kind, therefore in a truly scientific sense are not to be described as a cause."

In this ignorance as to the nature of the fundamental cause of disease resides the explanation for the lack of causal therapy, and for the want of correct prophylactic or preventive principles. This, also, is the explanation for the failure of symptomatic therapy. In opposition to the general mania for bacteriological causes of disease, how woefully few members of the medical profession occupy themselves with disposition to disease, with constitutional variations, and with problems arising from constitutional disturbances.

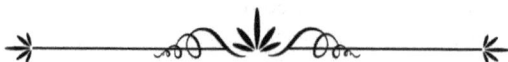

II.
SPECIALIZATION IS CAUSE
OF MEDICAL CHAOS

The reason for this fundamental ignorance is to be found in the point of view from which anatomy, physiology, pathology and therapy are taught. Let us compare the method of teaching anatomy in general use with the teaching of this subject when based upon physiological chemistry.

The method of teaching in general use is that founded by Galen, who has been dead almost two thousand years. He knew that a scaffolding is necessary in erecting a building, as his father was an architect. His method of teaching anatomy is based upon the skeleton. Thus vital knowledge of a living organism is to be sought in a heap of dead and glistening bones, in a skeleton. Could anything more absurd be conceived as scientific ? In fairness to Galen, let us admit that it was not absurd in his day—because chemistry was then unknown.

It is time for us to get away from dead bones. With the skeleton in the closet, what shall serve as the starting point of our anatomical studies? Whatever our starting point may be, we must view the body as a unit composed of a series of interdependent tissues and organs, as a chemical process, the result of which is the organization, agglomeration and diferrentiation of matter.

Viewed from this standpoint our study of anatomy must, as Hensel so well says: "Proceed from the mobile nerve substance, which lays alike the foundation and provides the form. That these two elements — the foundation and the form of our bodies—apparently opposed to each other—should, when viewed from a chemical standpoint, be found in hitherto unsuspected agreement, can only serve to support the view that all our bodily parts have their origin in one common fundamental material."

This view is generally admitted by scientists, but, thanks to the habit of following well-beaten trails, the proper conclusion to be drawn from it is rarely sensed by any of them. In other words, the habit of thinking of anatomy as nothing more than the study of a dead caricature of a man, a skeleton, is so strongly rooted in their minds that the idea of studying the subject from the point of view of the development and differentiation of protoplasmic material is given no thought at all.

A brief excursion into the domain of embryology would offer ample evidence of the folly of studying anatomy from a skeleton. It would reveal that the bones are not primary, but that the brain and the nervous system are first developed in the embryo. Indeed, the bones are formed very slowly by the deposition of calcium phosphate in glutinous cartilage, the process being incomplete even at the birth of the child. It is to be remarked that both the brain and the nervous tissues are built up of cells, and these cells, in turn, issue from the blood plasm. The point of departure for him who would understand how the body is built up, in short its anatomy and its physiology, must be the blood, not a bundle of bones !

In this connection I would cite the fact that the great Dubois-Reymond, while addressing one of his classes, said : "Gentlemen, we now proceed to the spleen. We know nothing of the spleen ; we pass to the liver."

Is it to be wondered at, then, that the medical profession of the world relies upon drugs and serums, upon scalpels, forceps, scissors, hammers, and saws to cure constitutional diseases? Want of basic knowledge must be covered with a multitude of instruments—a thermometer, spyghmograph, a plessimeter to tap the patient, a stethoscope to hear with, a catheter, bougies, and galvanic apparatus. But at the end, as a rule, Mother Earth must cover all !

The point of view from which scholastic physiology proceeds to the study of the body leads to the consideration of each process, of each organ and its function, independent of all others, as though they were things separate and apart from the chemico-electric process which animates the whole body. The fact is, physiology as taught in the schools nowadays has no basis on earth, but is a castle in the air. It is the failure of physiologists to stress the unity of the life process which is responsible, in part at least, for the development of symptomatic therapy. This failure to bear in mind the interdependence of all phases of the life process, the interdependence of the organs, leads a vast multitude of physicians to have recourse to antipyretics, febrifuges, cocaine, heroin, morphia, aspirin, and so on ad nauseam. It is also responsible for the production of another "unfailing serum" with the outbreak of each new epidemic. Humanity is to be given health with the aid of deadly drugs and putrefying matter!

It is more than fifty years since Prof. Jacob Moleschott called attention in unmistakable terms to the fact that the problem of health is bound up in the question, how shall we maintain the blood in a healthy bactericide state? But his words were uttered in vain, so far as the majority of physicians are concerned. The trinity on which they still rely consists of drugs, serums and knives !

In order that the reader may not think we minimize the effect of chemical discoveries upon the teaching of physiology in the medical departments of our colleges and universities, let us glance at the work of Albert P. Mathews, Professor of Physiological Chemistry in the University of Chicago, entitled : "Physiological Chemistry : A Textbook and Manual for Students." The edition in hand is the second, published in 1916, which contains more than a thousand pages. But all I can find devoted to the consideration of the function of the mineral elements in our food is comprised in the following quotation :

"Mineral substances are also necessary to life, and the result of keeping them out of the food is disastrous. In the perspiration and urine salts of various kinds are constantly being lost. Food as free as possible from mineral substances produced disturbances in the muscular system in Taylors' experiments on himself ; disturbances of the nervous system have also been noted by Forster. A sufficient supply of phosphates and calcium are essential to the development of the bones and teeth. Herbivorous animals constantly have a diet poor in sodium and relatively rich in potassium. Such animals require from time to time some sodium chloride added to their ration. Carnivorous animals require no salt, since the salts in their prey are about those of their own bodies."

These statements of Prof. Mathews occupy only eleven lines out of more than a thousand pages in his book. The following chapter of this work is devoted to the consideration of the function of the organic minerals in our foodstuffs, but it is impossible to refrain from making some comment on Prof. Mathews statements above quoted. We may ask, how much mineral matter is essential to the body ? It is reasonable, and scientific also, to conclude that if absence of mineral matter from foodstuff is dangerous, an insufficient quantity of them is also dangerous. We are told that minimizing the mineral content of his food produced muscular disturbance in Taylor's experiments on himself, and that Forster observed nervous disturbances under the same conditions, but we are not given so much as a hint as to the reason for these disturbances. No, Prof. Mathews seems to be utterly unaware of the physiological function of the mineral elements in the human system, and in this he is far from being alone.

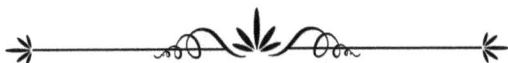

III.

THE FUNCTION OF ORGANIC MINERALS IN THE BODY

The material in this chapter was presented—in greater detail—to the chiefs of the Public Health Service, of the War Department, the Department of Agriculture, and to the Senators and Congressmen of the United States, in advance of the outbreak of the Spanish influenza pandemia, but the warning to be plainly read therein was ignored. This chapter represents an epitome of the most illuminating work to be found in the archives of physiological chemistry from the time of Johannes Mueller, a period of eighty years. A thorough understanding of the facts which follow would, if properly used in fighting the present pandemia, have saved hundreds of thousands of lives in this country alone.

There are sixteen chemical elements absolutely essential to healthy human life. In the composition of the human organism we constantly find these elements . Carbon, oxygen, hydrogen, nitrogen, iron, sulphur, phosphorus, chlorine, potassium, sodium, magnesium, calcium, manganese, fluorine, silicon and iodine.

Although chemical salts are only a small part of the material entering into the composition of our bodies, and are a very small item in our daily diet, their importance cannot be too strongly emphasized. They are the main sources for the development of electric-magnetic energy in the blood, and they perform other services. Whether you agree with me in thinking that they are the long-sought "vitamines"

/19

does not matter, but you must instantly agree that they are essential to perfect metabolism. It was Justus von Liebig who laid down the Law of the Minimum, according to which the absence of the tiniest essential ingredient necessary to the growth and functioning of a given tissue or organ will result in disease.

It goes without saying, of course, that no action in the world occurs without an impulse, hence the body must be given an impulse to grow. A series of chemical and physical facts indicate that phosphorus plays this vital part. The property of phosphoric acid of uniting with carburetted hydrogen to form carbonic acid and phosphuretted hydrogen is of fundamental importance, as phosphuretted hydrogen readily ignites on coming into contact with oxygen. Since the cerebrin consists of a combination of phosphoric acid with gelatine which contains ammonium, and with oleine, it is easy to infer that the light of the soul may be due to phosphoric acid in the nerves and still further the potassium phosphate forming the mineral basis of the muscles. Thus we come to the conclusion that the phosphates, combinations of phosphoric acid with basic substances, possess in general the property of imparting the true impulse to growth, the accumulation of organic matter.

The body, however, like every other structure, requires supports and props and, above all, a firm foundation on which to rest. Iron and lime, whose union is secured by their opposition to one another, bring into conjunction materials of contrary disposition for the creation of organic forms in the shape of plant and animal bodies.

The sulphuric compounds are all related, and yet all opposed, to the growth determining phosphoric compounds. All organic building material—all protein— contains phosphorus and sulphur in varying proportions, and all indications are that sulphur plays the part of a regulator in organic growth. This is a vital function as the human body requires a controlling factor to ensure definite stability to it, just as an engine requires a governor to regulate its pace. It is interesting to observe that normal blood contains about twice as many sulphates as phosphates. When there is great scarcity of sodium sulphate in the blood, abnormal growths develop from the phosphatic nerve tissues, and they continue to develop so long as the blood and lymph are deficient in sulphur, particularly in the sulphates. In the same manner that sulphuric acid controls and regulates the phosphoric acid of ammonium phosphate, so lime and magnesia act on this same ammonium phosphate.

When there is a deficiency of lime and magnesia in the system, phosphatic ammonium carbonate lodges in the gelatinous cartilage and stretches it, resulting in rickets. Such growth of cartilaginous tissues is controlled by lime and magnesia, as they change the pliant cartilage into bony barriers in which small particles of magnesia combine to produce phosphate of ammonium and magnesium which checks the further deposit of cartilage.

Lime and magnesia are indubitably quite as effective agents in the control of ammonia as sulphur is in the control of phosphorus. If we consider the minerals, leaving out of account chlorine and fluorine for the moment, as the foundation and mortar which gives stability to the vital machine, we find that this role is played by iron, manganese, potash, soda and silicic acid. Sulphur, because it possesses the property of becoming gaseous, is able to take part directly in the formation of albumen, that variable basis of body material, whereas all of the other mineral substances except silicic acid can only be assimilated in the form of salts, so-called binary compounds.

Normal blood albumen is essentially a compound of calcium and sodium into which iron and sulphur both enter. A deficiency of calcium commonly makes itself known by dental defects, just as lack of sulphur reveals itself by the falling out and poor growth of hair. Insufficiency of iron in the blood is evidenced, apart from lack of spirit, by paleness of face and blue lips ; insufficient sodium by glandular tumors and abnormal cartilaginous growths.

The entire amount of iron in the blood of an adult person is, on the average under normal conditions, four grams, as much as a nickel weighs. We may well judge that this amount is not sufficient to set the motive power of our bodies in action, if we overlook that complex factor the circulation of blood. The left side of the heart has the capacity of containing about six ounces of blood, and every heart beat drives this amount through the aorta. With seventy beats to the minute, twenty-five pounds of blood is pumped from the heart every minute. What is the result? That if the four grams of iron keep up such an incessant movement as to pass from the heart into the aorta sixty times an hour or 1,440 times in 24 hours, it may be asserted that in 24 hours 13 pounds of iron (that is, 1,440X4 grams) pass from the heart into the aorta. Can it be doubted, in view of this, that the iron serves to produce an electro-dynamic force?

In respect to the generation of electricity, it matters not whether there be an entirely new supply of iron passing a given point, or whether the same iron pass that point anew each minute. Two factors work together in the circulation of the blood, namely, the active attraction of nerve tissue and the passive susceptibility of the blood contents to that attraction. Faraday has conclusively shown that blood is magnetic in character because of the iron it contains. If four grams of iron is the normal quantity in the blood, it is clear that the reduction of this amount, say by two grams, will lessen its susceptibility and slacken its circulation. The electrical nerve ends will then strain in vain for the electricity which the blood current should yield, and the result will be neuralgia.

It is the magnetic iron in haemoglobin which makes every sort of nervous function possible, in the cerebral (brain) and in the sympathetic (intestinal) tracts, and since it is thus made clear that intellectual activity on the one hand and breathing and digestion and excretion on the other are dependent on the iron content of the blood, we must also recognize that, as iron attends every nerve action, the secretion of urine too takes place under the influence of haemoglobin. Insofar as haemoglobin hastens the departure of the excrementitious matter in urine out of the system, there is a daily loss of iron in the urine. This loss in the form of urohaematin may total four centigrams, or a hundredth part of our supply.

This loss of iron if not replaced by eating suitable food will soon make itself felt. In the course of a day the reduction by four centigrams will diminish the energy of nervous activity about 1440 times the apparent loss, so that even a four weeks fever, during which no meat is eaten may completely exhaust the strength of an individual. Moreover, iron conditions bodily warmth as it combines with oxygen in a higher and a lower degree. In the lungs it is highly oxidized by the respired oxygen, but in contact with the nerve ends it gives itself only to a part of the oxygen present, and burns a certain portion of the lecithin to water, carbonic acid and phosphates, thus creating body warmth to a considerable extent.

In response to the chemical consumption of lecithin a new oil flows down the axis cylinders of the nerve fibrils, which are arranged like lamp wicks. The duration of the flow of this oil is, on the average, about eighteen hours. When the cerebro-spinal nerves refuse longer to perform their function fatigue and sleep ensue, and the current of blood leaves the brain and seeks the intestines. While the cerebro-spinal system rests, the sympathetic system takes up its task of directing the renewal of tissues and supplying the nerve sheaths through the lymph vessels, which draw their material from the digestive canal, with a new supply of phosphatic oil. Thus the brain and spinal nervous system are prepared for another day's work. For the fulfillment of these processes, the magnetic blood current forms the intermediary.

The presence of formic and acetic acid supplies the blood with fresh electricity to stimulate the nerves. "Under normal conditions," says Julius Hensel, "this function is assigned to the spleen. This organ takes the part of a rejuvenating influence in the body in the manner of a relay station, and does so by virtue of an invisible but significant device. In every other region of the body the hairlike terminals of the arteries which branch out from the heart, merge directly in the tiny tubes (capillaries) of the veins, which lead back to the heart again ; in the spleen this is not the case. Here rather the arteries end suddenly when they have diminished to a diameter of one one-hundred-and-fortieth of an inch and end in a bulb (the Malpighian bodies). Under such circumstances the sudden stoppage, particularly the impact of the magnetic blood stream against the membrane of a Malpighian body, exemplifies the physical law of the induction of electricity, in accordance with which the blood that enters the spleen is changed into plasma and exudes through the membranes of the Malpighian bodies. The event indicates some fluidity of the red blood cells, which is a change affected in the body by the impact of electric sparks, and one which electrical therapy also brings about locally to prevent increase in the solid constituents of the blood."

The numerous Malpighian bodies in the spleen act as so many electrical conductors, and the product of their electrical activity is found in the formic and acetic acid of the fluid plasma which filters through the Malpighian corpuscles and supplies the acid tissues of the spleen (pulpa splenica). These acids are the electrolytic division products of lecithin. In the splenic pulp arise the capillaries of the splenic veins whose acid blood is carried directly to the liver, where certain cells formed like galvanic elements possess the property, through the electrical action of formic and acetic acid, of extracting from blood albumen the opposite of acids, namely, alkaline bile. The normal functioning of the liver, therefore, is dependent upon that of the spleen, and since the bile produced by the liver goes to aid the digestive activity of the duodenum, disturbances of digestion must result when the quality of the bile is inferior.

One of the substances contained in bile, lecithin, is of wide importance. When it was referred to a moment ago, I spoke only of its individual chemical nature as a fat in combination with ammonium phosphate, as by so doing I avoided error in connection with its apparently complicated formula, which includes glycerophosphoric acid, trimethylamin, palmitic and stearic acids. As it is a fatty substance, the only question that arises is—what does it contain besides fat ? This may be answered by a process of subtraction :

$2 (C_{21} H_{42} O_4) C_{42} H_{84} O_8$ which represents tallow or stearate of glycerine. Lecithin, $C_{42} H_{84} O_9$ NP differs from this only by a larger amount of ONP. The significance of this difference becomes clear when two atoms of water are added. Then ammonium phosphate $PO_3 H_4$ N is formed. The two atoms of water needed for the condensation of the ammonium phosphate from the stearate are obtained by separating them away from two of glycerine.

The bile contains lecithin in a partially oxidized form. The chemical 'remainders" are biliverdin and cholesterin. The latter when normal has, as you know, the power to neutralize snake venoms and other poisons, and thus acts as a natural anti-toxin. In addition, the bile contains combinations of stearine with gelatine and with carbonate and sulphate of sodium, which theoretical chemists believe are twin compounds of glycocholate and taurocholate. These fatty compounds depend upon stearine partly oxidized, that is, deprived of a certain number of atoms of hydrogen.

As the compounds of fatty acid with ammoniacal blood gelatine and sodium carbonate, the ingredients of the bile also develop into a peculiar soap. In the economy of the body the bile acts as a soap. When it is discharged into the duodenum, it changes the fats into so fine an emulsion (chyle) that the microscopically fine drops of fat may be drawn into the orifices of the lymph canals and conveyed to the circulatory system, and the cleavage products of albumen produced by gastric digestion, the peptones (leucin and tyrosin) are carried along with them for the renewal of tissue cells consumed in respiration.

If a soda soap is requisite for the purpose just stated, it follows that soda in the food is essential, as otherwise the supply of soda in the blood albumen cannot be renewed, and the bile cannot get its necessary supply of soda from blood albumen devoid of soda. Consequently, the entire nutritive process is dependent upon bile, and the bile cannot properly perform its function if denied soda.

In addition to carbonate of sodium, especially the hydrocarbonate known as glycolate, the bile apparently contains ammonium sulphate combined with hydrocarbon (taurin) ; but this results from the transposition of sodium sulphate and gelatine. Gelatine contains six atoms of hydrocarbon joined with two of ammonium carbonate, a group which is separable by chemical action into five of carburetted hydrogen with ammonium carbonate (leucin or gelatine milk), $C_5 H_{10} C_{O2} NH_3$ and into one of carburetted hydrogen with ammonium carbonate (glycin or gelatine sugar) $CH_2 CO_2 NH_3$. This latter substance, gelatine sugar, is not produced in the liver, as it exists already in the blood gelatine. In an isolated condition it has the property, in virtue of its ammonical acids and its carbonic acid bases and, therefore, of both combined, its salts, of producing chemical fixation. This property is conveyed to the undivided blood gelatine in which the gelatine sugar is contained intramolecularly.

Since normal blood albumen is inconceivable without sulphur, it is absolutely essential, in accordance with our knowledge of the constituents of the bile and their origin, that our nutriment should contain a sufficiency of sodium sulphate, if normal

/23

blood serum is to be produced. The use of pepsin for this purpose cannot serve nature's purpose, as it contains neither sodium carbonate nor sodium sulphate. Our blood must be given a fresh and sufficient supply of sodium carbonate and sodium sulphate via our food, if it is to produce normal bile and supply the requisites of normal nutrition.

It is erroneously held that sodium sulphate is simply a laxative, even Borner's "Royal Medical Calendar" so classifies it. Often it discharges this function, it is true, in concentrated solution (one to five). But it is an important ingredient of healthy blood albumen (one to one thousand), and in this proportion assists in the formation of normal bile.

The blood of the Caucasian race is found to contain about ten parts of salt to the thousand, and this proportion of salt denotes firm tissue material. If the quantity of salt in the blood is diminished, the bi-concave red blood cells swell to a spherical form from access of water and lose their ability to unite for the production of connective tissue. Moreover, to the extent salt in the blood cells is decreased, the connective tissue and muscle and tendon substance absorb water and the tissues become spongy, especially in the kidneys, so that the thinned blood albumen seeps through (urea albumen).

Phosphate of potassium is the mineral basis of muscle tissue, phosphate of lime with a small amount of magnesium phosphate the basis of bones, and phosphate of ammonium the basis of nervous tissue. There is a sufficient quantity of phosphate in all healthy foods. When the milk fed to nurslings, however, is greatly thinned with water instead of firm muscle fibre and solid lymph glands, we find loose and spongy tissues. This is a scrofulous condition.

In the formation of healthy bones and teeth, calcium fluoride is essential. It is insoluble in plain water, but is made soluble by the aid of the glycocoll in blood gelatine and changed into ammonium fluoride. It appears in this form in the cartilaginous matter of the eye lenses, and lack of calcium fluoride in the food results in the clouding of these lenses.

Silicic acid is not only indispensible to the growth of hair, but it forms a direct connection between blood and nerve tissues. It is found in birds eggs, both in the white and the yolk. It is a conservator of heat and electricity, as it is a good insulator. It also possesses eminent antiseptic qualities. Its mere presence in the intestinal canal, even its simple passage through the canal, conserves the electrical activity of the intestinal nerves and thus influences the whole sympathetic nervous system.

This brief review, cursory as it is, of the function of the minerals in the renewal of substances undergoing tissue change, makes it clear that our daily food must contain a sufficient quantity of them if healthy metabolism is to be maintained.

Chemically considered the human body is one individual whole, its characteristic chemical basis being gelatine. Lieut. C. E. McDonald, U. S. A. Medical Corps, recognized this when he recently wrote: "The similarity of chemical compositions explains why, when any particular region falls a prey to chemical decomposition, others quickly become affected."

Oxygen gas is the medium through which chemical combustion is carried on in the body for the purpose of preparing materials to enter into its composition. The mineral salts already named not only form the solid basis of the various tissue but also serve as conductors or insulators of electricity in the body. The absence of one of them for a protracted period is sufficient to explain widespread degeneration in the system.

In view of the fact that these various minerals play an indispensible part in healthy metabolism it is imperative that a sufficiency of them should be applied in proper proportion in our food daily—if we desire to retain or restore health to the body.

Indeed, the instincts of both animals and human beings leads them under certain conditions right back to the earth and its lesson. Note the avidity with which hens confined in arid runs devoid of vegetation, worms, insects, and small stones devour a compound of lime and ground bones and oyster shells. Observe a child whose ration is deficient in mineral elements eating egg shells, wall plaster, chalk and other earthy substances. What do these things mean? Nothing more than this : both chicken and child express a natural craving for the essential elements to build bone and form the basis for the tissue.

I have stressed the important part the minerals play in both the vegetable and animal kingdom for the purpose of stressing our great need of more of them in our daily diet, and I may add that this is equally as true in the case of those we call healthy as of those who are diseased. No matter how carefully the diet may be regulated as regards the quantity of protein and carbohydrates and fats, and the ratio between them, healthy metabolism is impossible without a sufficiency of the essential minerals.

In view of the facts with regard to the function of these minerals, it is indisputably true that a ration is physiologically inefficient if it does not contain a sufficiency of them in proper proportion. Moreover, this is trebly true in the case of those whose constitution has been weakened by loss of blood from wounds, by shell shock and trench fever, and of those here at home whose nerve tissue has been degenerated and whose blood has been weakened by anxiety and the strain of unwonted manual labor. The last consideration applies with especial force to the multitudes of women who have entered industry as manual laborers. What kind of offspring can we expect from these people whose plasma is thus degenerated? The children are the citizens of the future, and even before they are born we must plan for their health.

I am the last person in the world to deny that wonderful progress is made in surgery every day, and the last to fail to applaud its successful efforts, but you know quite as well as I do that in ninety out of one hundred cases recovery involves exhaustion of the patient's reserve energy. Moreover, when the reserve energy has already been drawn upon almost to the point of exhaustion, no matter how successful the operation may be, the recovery of the patient is a very doubtful quantity. The first requisite in all surgical cases, as also in all anaemic and neurasthenic cases, is to restore metabolism to its normal condition and thus help the patient to regain his reserve energy in order to prevent the collapse of the whole fabric.

It is indubitably true that healthy metabolism and the restoration of reserve energy depends upon the organism being given the requisite quantity of the sixteen essential elements of organic life in easily digestible and assimilable form. I have not entered into a full discussion of the various aspects of my method, but have confined myself to consideration of the basic principles underlying it. Neither have I attempted to show how these different minerals will serve as regenerative agents in different dysaemic conditions. I am prepared to discuss the matter from both of these viewpoints, however, and—more than that—I am ready to practically demonstrate the soundness of my theories, when given an opportunity under proper conditions to do so.

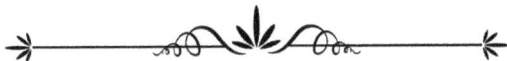

IV.
MEDICAL DIAGNOSIS AND SYMPTOMATIC THERAPY

The description of influenza which follows is from the pen of Prof. George Kuhnemann, an authority on practical and differential diagnosis. But I am constrained to remark in advance, a list of symptoms, with the order of their probable appearance, and possible complications, is not a diagnosis of a disease in the sense that the underlying cause is revealed. Before a successful attempt can be made to diagnose a disease in this sense, we must recognize that both the objective and the subjective symptoms are but the reflex of an underlying cause, and we must seek that cause. Only when we know the cause of a disease are we in a position to tell what it is.

The facts cited in the previous chapter afford ample proof of the correctness of what has just been said. But most physicians are not familiar with the chemico-physiological process of the body as a whole, and in consequence have been content to ascertain and suppress individual symptoms with the aid of drugs. The failure of these efforts in connection with the Spanish influenza has been confessed by some of the leading medical men.

As careful consideration of all the symptoms of the disease and the effect of trying to remove those symptoms with the aid of drugs, can only serve to emphasize the accuracy of my diagnosis and the soundness of my method of treating it. I am giving Prof. Kuhnemann's description in full :

"Fever is always present," Prof. Kuhnemann says, "but not of any certain type. At times, after short periods of Apyrexie there is a rise in temperature, sometimes swelling of the spleen. There is no characteristic change in the urine ; sometimes Albuminuria. There is an inclination to perspire freely ; consequently Miliaria is often present ; also Herpes, less frequently other Exanthema, Petechien. The mucous membranes are inclined to hemorrhage (Epistaxis, Hematemesis, Menorrhagia, Abortion). "Complications and after effects" he lists as : "1. On the part of the respiratory system : Croupose and Broncho-pneumonia of atypical progress (atypical fever of protracted course, relatively strong Dyspnoe, Cyanosis, feeble pulse) and high mortality; after effects serous or mattery Pleuritis, Lung abscesses, Phthisis. 2. On the part of the circulatory system: Myocarditis, Endocarditis, Thrombose. 3. On the part of the digestive tract: Chronic stomach and intestinal catarrh, Dyspepsia. 4. On the part of the nervous system: Any form of Neuralgia, Paralysis, Neuritis, Psychosis, etc. 5. On the part of the sense organs: Otitis media, Nephritis and Muscular Rheumatism are observed. Influenza aggravates any case of sickness, especially lung trouble.

"Aetiologie : The influenza bacillus (found in blood and excrement) is to be regarded as the cause. The malady is highly contagious. Period of incubation given as, from two to seven days. Runs its course in one to two weeks, recovery as a rule favorable; though convalescence is often protracted. Unfavorable results are brought on through complications, most often by Pneumonia.

"Diagnosis: Easily determined during an epidemic or marked symptoms. The catarrhal form of influenza differs from simple catarrh of the mucous membranes of the respiratory tract through the presence of nervous symptoms and a more abrupt beginning. The symptoms may be similar to those of Measles or Abdominal typhus. In each case, complications with Pneumonia must be considered.

"The proof of the presence of the Influenza bacillus," he concludes, "is of little value in the diagnosis and differential diagnosis in medical practice as the bacillus cannot be distinguished with enough accuracy through the microscopic examination, which must be a very minute culture proceeding." The words of a great poet characterize the learned professor, and most medical men perfectly: "He holds the parts within his hand, but lacks the mental grasp of all."

So much for the symptomatic description of the disease ; now we will glance briefly at the train of symptoms and locate their individual causes :

The ever present fever is due to stagnation of the blood. This is discussed somewhat at length later. Swelling of the spleen caused by catabolism of the Malpighian bodies. Albuminuria the result of cold in the Plexus renalis ; Perspiration due to numbness in nerve fibrils. The inclination of the mucous membranes to Hemorrhage is explained by congestion of blood in the capillaries, which is due to lack of vigor in the nerve fibrils: When the nerve fibrils fail to act, the capillary circulation stops and the blood overloaded with carbonic acid presses against the walls until they burst.

The complications and after effects are explained in the following manner:

Complications in the respiratory system are all due to failure to properly treat the acute stage of the disease, and where the resistance of the patient has been sapped they usually end lethally—that is, in death. The complications which appear in the circulatory system are subject to the same explanation as fever. The digestive complications are to be explained by impairment of metabolism brought on by the loss of energy by the Vagus nerve. Those complications arising in the nervous system are explainable as consequences of the degeneration of the whole Vagus tract. Sensory complications are due to the disease finding lodgement in the "minoris resistentia," the point of least resistance of the patient.

In the light of the foregoing explanation of the meaning of the various symptoms of influenza, it should be clear that their cause is deep seated, that it is spread over a large part of the organism. But the regular practitioner of medicine will, ninety-nine times out of a hundred, treat the disease in the manner indicated below.

The fever he will immediately seek to suppress with the aid of one of the hundred or more febrifuges; i. e. a drug whose purpose is to allay or dispel it.

In catarrhal respiratory complications, the doctor will prescribe Dover powder (Opium and Ipecac) (two rank poisons) Aspirin, Nitr. of Bismuth, Morphine Muriate, Laudanum, etc., for the stomach and bowels; Tincture of Laudanum (opiate), Morphine Muriate, Syrup of Ipecac, Codein (opiate) Belladonna, etc. for the bronchial tubes and lungs. No, he will not give them all at once !

In cases where nervous complications are grave, the doctor will, as a general rule, seek to allay the pain by giving one or more of the following drugs: Nitr. Bromide, Sulfonal, Sulphate of Sublimat, Chloroform, Hyosciam, Morphine Muriate, Extract Opii, Chloral Hydrate, or any one of a great list of others. They are intended, of course, to allay pain, but the fact that they narcotize and paralyze the nerves, and therefore hinder metabolism and assist the process of catabolism is lost sight of.

In cases where the influenza takes the dyspeptic or gastro-intestinal form, the list of drugs cited in connection with the discussion of the catarrhal respiratory phase of the disease will be used, being varied according to the whim of the physician in charge.

The utter futility of this symptomatic therapy, to call it by no harsher name, will be perfectly apparent to anyone capable of thinking for himself after he reads the description of the disease and the course of treatment recommended by the present writer.

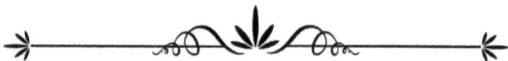

V.
THE WANDERING ROOT OF
THE INFLUENZA

The symptomatic description of the disease given by Prof. Kuhnemann in the last chapter was summed up by him in the statement that the bacillus found in the blood and excrement of the patient is to be regarded as its cause. But, he adds that the bacillus cannot be observed with a microscope accurately enough to be of much use in making the diagnosis. It is to be noted that he does not flatly say the bacillus is the cause, but only says it is to be regarded as the cause.

This is the last word medical science has to say with respect to the basic cause of influenza ; the bacillus is to be regarded as its cause. But why should we regard the bacillus as the cause? To arbitrarily regard the bacillus as cause is to beg the question. It is clear, however, that medical science has no idea of how to ascertain the cause. Whatever else it may be, viewing the bacillus as the cause is unscientific. What a thing is and does, that is what science seeks to explain. Scientific knowledge is based upon facts, and. deals with laws, but has no relation to dogmatic opinions.

As a matter of fact, all the evidence of Prof. Kuhnemann's diagnosis, every symptom he lists, points unerringly to something beyond the bacillus as the primary cause of the disease. When the basis of those symptoms is explained, the medical profession would, indeed, be hard put to disprove that the bacillus is a result of the disease, instead of its cause.

The symptoms so fully described by Prof. Kuhnemann, and observed by all physicians coming in contact with the disease, all occur in those regions where the

Vagus (Wandering) or Pneumogastric nerve functions. It will be wise, therefore, to observe the course of this nerve, to remark its connections, and note its functions. The facts thus gathered may be of use to us in tracing the objective symptoms of influenza to their source. In the last analysis, of course, the bodily processes are a unit, and this must be borne in mind if we are not to be led astray by appearances, by objective symptoms.

The functions of the *Vagus* may be roughly divided into two classes, physiological and psychic. They are listed in advance of the discussion of the character of this nerve, for the purpose of emphasizing the striking parallel between its functions and the symptoms of influenza. Broadly stated, its physiological function is to regulate breathing, tasting, swallowing, satisfaction of hunger, digestion, etc., and its failure to properly control those functions finds expression in coughing, choking, or indigestion, or vomiting, with acute pain, or in a combination of two or more of them. Its psychic function includes assisting in the expression of shame, desire, disgust, grief, anguish, etc.

This Vagus nerve, like a wandering vagabond, is creating a great deal of disturbance, and in order that we may understand him we will let science describe him for us. This is the exact description: *Vagus* or Pneumogastric nerve (tenth cranial) ; function—sensation and motion; originates in the floor of the fourth ventricle (the space which represents the primitive cavity of the hind-brain ; it has the pons and oblongata in front, while the cerebellum lies dorsal), and is distributed through the ear, pharynx, larynx, lungs, esophagus, and stomach ; possesses the following branches— auricular, pharyngeal, superior and inferior laryngeal, cardiac, pulmonary, esophageal, gastric, hepatic, communicating, meningeal.

The physician and the interested lay reader should turn back and read Prof. Kuhnemann's description of influenza in the light of this exposition of the ramifications and the functions of the Vagus nerve.

II.

So that the deductions to be drawn from the operation of the *Vagus* may be indisputable, let us glance at the manner in which nerve tissue is formed in the first instance and observe what occurs in nerve metabolism.

An inherent impulse in the ovum (protoplasm; egg cell) serves to separate the albuminous substance into groups of an opposite nature. Water is chemically separated from one portion, which results in thickening the albumen from which it was extracted, while the liberated water aids in liquifying another portion of the albuminous matter. Thus arises, on one side slender threads termed fibrine or filaments, and on the other appears lymph liquor, which receives the particles of salts freed from the filaments during their chemical separation. When the fibrine and lymph are organized from the protoplasm, the remaining albumen is absolutely unchanged and ready to furnish material for the growth of either.

It is the function of salts to increase the electrical tension of the lymph. All salts possess the property of being electrically positive or negative. The more concentrated a saline solution, the greater its electrical energy.

That the function of the lymph is to assist in the formation and nutrition of the nerves is apparent when the nature of lymph and the composition of nerve substances are compared. The contrast which exists between fibrine and lymph, and the similarity of lymph to nerve marrow, when taken together, justify the conclusion that the nerve substance, lecithin, was formed from lymph in the first instance.

The whole process of life consists of an electro-chemical combustion. This is clearly shown in the case of lecithin, which serves to control both motion and sensation. In the presence of oxygen it burns up, forming a new chemical combination, and throwing off minute quantities of carbonic acid and water in the process. Every movement and process, both voluntary and involuntary, and every thought and emotion, depends upon oxidation, which consumes muscular tissue and nerve substance.

The greater our physical exertion the more muscular tissue must be consumed. The higher our emotional state, the more we think, the greater must be the quantity of nerve substance burned up. All of the substance burned up in labor, in worry and thought, must be replaced or the flame will flicker out !

The metabolism of muscular tissue is beside the point at this moment. We are concerned here with nerve metabolism alone. This occurs in the following manner: In response to the demand for new material created by the chemical combustion of lecithin, new oil flows down the axis and cylinders of the nerve fibrils, which are arranged somewhat in the manner of lamp wicks. The average duration of the flow of this oil is about eighteen hours. When the cerebro-spinal nerves refuse to perform their function any longer, because the supply of oil is running low, fatigue and sleep ensue, and the blood descends from the brain to the intestines. Thus the cerebro-spinal system is permitted to relax and rest. In the meantime the sympathetic nervous system has taken up the task of directing the renewal of worn tissues, which draw their supply of necessary materials from the digestive canal, with a new supply of phosphatic oil. For the carrying out of these processes, which prepare the brain and spinal nerve system to perform another day's work, the magnetic blood current forms the intermediary.

It follows inexorably that (1) a radical change in our diet may result in giving us an insufficient supply of the various elements necessary for the production of lecithin in the proper quantity; (2) physical labor to which we are unaccustomed may involve a greater consumption of nerve substance as well as muscular tissue, and then our normal diet will not be able to supply our need; (3) or a long continued emotional tension may affect at once our appetite and our digestion while it continues to burn up our nerves.

III.

In discussing the causes of disease Julius Hensel lays great stress upon the emotions. He goes so far as to say that they "undoubtedly occupy the first place amongst the factors causing disease, and we must not evade the consideration of them. We shall find that their action also amounts to an electro-chemical process." I would not for one instant be understood to hold that the emotions alone are sufficient to explain the origin of disease—far from it. There are other factors—sometimes they are dominant—diet, nature of occupation, changes in the weather, climate.

Insofar as the present pandemia is concerned, however, there can be no doubt in the mind of any person who is willing to think the matter out for himself in the light of the electro-chemical nature of life, that the emotional stress incident to the war, plus dietetic upheavals, offer an explanation of it.

It is to be remembered that the Spanish influenza arose in Europe as an epidemic, in 1917, and in the course of a few months it had become pandemic.

The outbreak of the war in 1914 shook the whole civilized world to its very foundations, emotionally. More than that, it upset the international relations of people in every part of the globe. It forced the peoples of Europe to go on a new ration. Some twenty million men had to shoulder arms and march away to the battlefields, leaving behind them mothers, wives, children, relatives. Soon the roar of Mars echoed and reechoed around the world.

There is no need of entering into a detailed description of the emotional state of the peoples directly concerned in the war or of those immediately adjacent to the war zones; it was an emotional conflagration, a holocaust of hate and horror, of fear and anguish.

The *Vagus* nerve, as stated a moment ago, is concerned with the expression of these very emotions. In consequence of the high tension of the emotions it was consumed at an alarming rate. It is almost incredible that this fact has been given no thought whatever in connection with the spread of Spanish influenza !

The diet of the peoples most closely affected by the war was not only greatly changed, but also much curtailed. There was a veritable flood of substitutes for the usual foods of these people. I am not discussing whether the nutritive value of these substitutes was high or low, but I want to make the point that they involved a dietetic and digestive revolution. The curtailment of the quantity of foods which the people were in the habit of consuming daily is of very great significance. Both of these facts together show that a fresh burden was added for already overburdened bodies to carry.

It is absolutely essential to the maintenance of physical normality, to health, that the metabolic process shall keep pace with the catabolic. In plain words, the body must be given enough fresh nutritive material to replace what has been burnt up in labor, in thought or emotion.

Very shortly after the beginning of the war, for two obvious reasons, namely, the shipping situation or lack of contact with outside countries, and especially those overseas, and with the withdrawal of vast numbers of men from agriculture and industry, the price of fats, eggs, flour, etc., began to soar ever higher. In the course of a little more than two years many of these essential foodstuffs were fetching practically their weight in gold on the continent of Europe.

Moreover, the withdrawal of millions of men from productive labor in order to fight imposed upon those remaining behind, both women and men, the necessity of carrying on the work of supplying the fighters with food and munitions. Indeed, even a multitude of children had to participate in this labor.

The nature of most of this work was nerve racking, to say the least of it, and much of it was dangerous in a high degree—the making of high-power explosives and deadly gases, for instance—thus adding to the nerve strain.

The details as to this phase of the situation can be readily filled in by any well-informed and thoughtful person. Hence, I will not catalog them here. Shell shock, trench fever, etc. are known to all.

It is impossible in passing, however, not to stress the fact that the effect of unwonted manual labor, or manual labor of a type with which they were utterly unfamiliar, upon the sensitive organism in the case of a multitude of women was bound to be disastrous. This was, of course, doubly assured by the fact that their nourishment was insufficient for their needs, or of an improper nature.

Instead of a curtailed diet—and it was curtailed both as regards variety of items and quantity—this was just the time when, because of greatly increased combustion of lecithin and muscle tissue, there should have been an increase in the food ration.

In the case of a great many women—mothers, wives, sweethearts of the fighting men—their emotional tension, their fears, worries, and very often their anguish, was so great as to diminish their appetites and upset their digestions.

The effect of this emotional conflagration could not be other than the depletion of the Vagus, the reduction of the vital resistance, and the preparation of the soil for an epidemic, aye, for a pandemia of influenza, and all sorts of constitutional disturbances.

If it be said that the war was confined to Europe and that but few of the warriors came from abroad, the answer is that the economic and emotional life of the entire world was convulsed and upset by it. Not only economically, but even more important, emotionally, the effects of the war were felt in the home of millions of people in this country.

There is no need of laboring the point, as he who is not blind must see the relation between the emotional stress of the war and the pandemia of Spanish influenza.

The matter has been discussed in broad outlines herein because there is not time to enter details at every point. This is an occasion where haste is justified, as the sacrifice of life goes on unchecked while the nature and cause of the pandemia are not understood.

IV.

We have just seen the effect of malnutrition and strenuous labor and protracted emotional tension upon the electromagnetic forces of the Vagus, as well as upon the rest of the human organism. Disturbing influences, as we know, may abnormally increase or decrease the positive or negative electrons. The effect of decrease of their number will be apparent in a moment.

When the slowly vibrating negative outnumber the rapidly vibrating positive electrons, the electronic vibration of the whole body is lowered. The result is that we become depressed, feel weak and tired, possess little bodily warmth. Our metabolism is upset, falls far below normal, and the skin becomes pale, because of the morbid action set up in the mucous membrane by the overplus of negative electrons. Catarrh arises. This is the ground in which negative diseases thrive : Influenza, nervous debility, anaemia, cholera, diptheria, etc.

/34

The proper therapeutic method to use in the treatment of negative diseases, particularly in the treatment of influenza, has already been indicated in the course of this discussion, but it will form the subject of the next and concluding chapter, where it will be shown in detail.

VI.

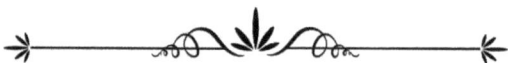

THERAPEUTIC MEASURES FOR THE INFLUENZA

Influenza is a negative disease, as we have seen ; a member of the catarrhal group of affections. After careful consideration of all aspects of its origin and development, I am of the opinion that it would be more accurate to name this disease *Panasthenia* : general loss of vitality.

Insofar as prophylactic measures are concerned, we may sum them up very briefly : Keep your head cool, physically and mentally ; your feet warm, the bowels regular, the pores open, and breathe plenty of fresh air. Eat enough wholesome food to satisfy your appetite. In short, keep your metabolism (the process of discarding worn-out matter and replacing it with fresh nutritive material) in good order.

But if for any reason you experience a chill these days, go to bed at once as a precaution. Put on a warm abdominal pack, drink a good hot lemonade, sweetened, and strengthened (if possible) with some good old rum or grape brandy. Then relax, forget your personal troubles and go to sleep. Nine times out of ten, you will awaken with a moist feeling all over the body. Take a warm sponge bath on arising, dress warmly, and remain at home for a few days. Thus all danger may be averted. This course is easy to follow. Ignorance of it has cost a great many people their life !

In case you were belated in commencing this preventive treatment, you may be the one out of ten who does not awaken with that fine warm feeling after the first use of the abdominal pack. Remember the first injunction, keep your head cool and don't worry. Repeat the pack treatment in the evening, and if possible keep it on all night. When you awaken in the morning you will feel as though your body had lost a dead weight during the night, as, in fact, it will have : For the pores of the skin, thanks to the pack, will throw off a mass of impurities. Thus you will save your lungs, bronchial tubes, kidneys, etc., from being overloaded with self-created poisons called auto-toxins. In other words, you will have assisted nature in carrying on the process of metobolism in your body. Only in rare cases, if this treatment is started soon enough, will it be necessary for the patient to remain in bed several days. In such cases, of course, modification of the treatment must be adjusted to the individual case.

As very few people know how to make or apply the abdominal pack properly, I will give an illustration of it and some instructions for making it.

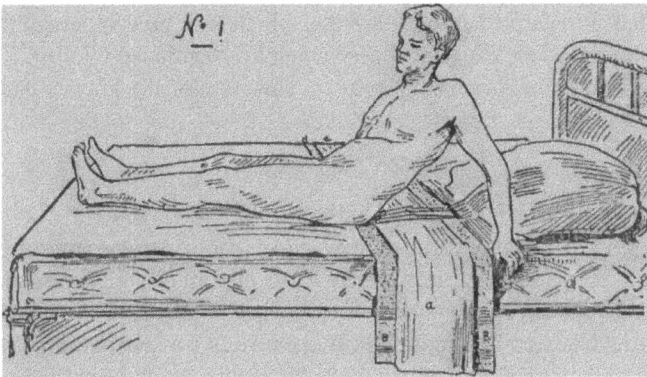

The abdominal pack should reach from the breast nipples to below the hips. It is made from a clean piece of woolen cloth or a blanket, which must be wide enough to reach from the nipples to a point just below the hips, and long enough to go around the body and fold over the front. In addition, two or three coarse linen towels which have been frequently laundered, or suitable pieces of linen cloth, and a few safety pins are needed.

Sometimes the pack has to be made narrower so as to cover only the stomach and belly (7 to 8 inches wide) and the woolen part must be folded accordingly. For children a towel, as a rule, will do nicely. In the case of infants, a properly folded piece of old linen will serve. The linen as well as the woollen material must be measured and properly folded in advance, so that the patient will not have to wait too long while the pack is being put on. The cut shows how the pack is to be put on an adult patient.

The towel or linen cloth is dipped into vinegar-water, (composed of two parts water and one part vinegar), the temperature of which should range from 90 to 100 degrees Fahrenheit, then wrung out and placed on the woollen material in such a position as to leave a margin of two or three inches of woollen goods at the top and bottom. The pack is now placed around the back of the patient, who sits up in bed, or is held up by an assistant. His shirt is lifted up and he lies down on the moist linen, which must be quickly folded up over the abdomen and covered with the woolen cloth. The latter is then pinned together at the middle and top and bottom with safety pins. The shirt is pulled down and the patient carefully covered. This pack must be applied speedily to prevent the patient from being chilled.

A similar pack should be applied to the feet and a hot water bottle placed against them.

These packs can be allowed to remain on the patient from one to two hours, depending entirely upon how he feels. When he becomes restless, however, immediately remove the packs.

Thus far we have dealt with the question of augmenting the electro-magnetic force of the body, which the packs are intended to accomplish by the increase of bodily heat and the stimulation of the capillary circulation. It may be asked why vinegar should be used for this purpose. The acetic acid of vinegar is absorbed through the pores and transformed into an acetate, which will prevent coagulation of the blood. This removes the cause of those symptoms mentioned by Prof. Kuhnemann in connection with the circulatory system. Thus one of the gravest dangers is removed.

II.

It may appear paradoxical, but fever accompanies severe attacks of negative as well as positive diseases. But we must know, first of all, the nature of fever, and the variations in its development in different types of physique and mentality, if we are not to grievously err in handling it. It operates like a fire, burning up infectious matter. Unless the nerve fibrils are already paralyzed, an evil smelling perspiration which follows the fever carries off the auto-toxins through the pores. In any case, it is the duty of the physician to control and guide the fever.

What shall be done to control fever in a given case depends not only upon the temperature, but on the physique and temperament of the patient also. It may be said that people of a calm, phlegmatic disposition will not suffer from very high fever, except in the case of serious complications. Those of quick, volatile temperament, and most children, on the other hand, often suffer from high fever without serious complications. It is unnecessary to argue that different treatment is called for in each of these cases.

The normal temperature for human beings varies between 98.6 and 99.5, and fever is recognized the moment the thermometer records 100.4 F, according to the usual medical diagnosis, and an effort is made immediately to restore the temperature to its normal level. But this practice is in flat contradiction to the teachings of physiological chemistry. Viewing the problem from the latter point of view, it does not follow that the fever should at once be reduced. Not at all. The disposition of the patient and the nature of the disease, as already indicated, must both enter into the calculation as to what is best to do.

The speedy reduction of a fever involves lowering the excitement present in the internal organs of the patient, and also the complete stoppage of a process of combustion which is destroying infectious matter.

In the case of a physically strong and phlegmatic patient, the speedy reduction of the fever is not only permissible, but is desirable. Such a patient can stand, and indeed requires, the reduction of the internal excitement. But in the case of a person of weak physique and nervous temperament, the reduction of the fever must proceed slowly, as the swift reduction of it would be dangerous.

The fever should always be reduced in accordance with the strength of the patient, never faster or more than he can stand, if extreme nervous irritation, which has caused the death of countless human beings, is not to follow. It is better, therefore, to leave a nervous patient's fever undisturbed while we seek to strengthen him so that he can overcome the fever without outside aid.

For this purpose I recommend simple ablutions, and in some cases the application of the abdominal pack already described. In addition, the vigor of the patient is to be increased by giving him alternately Dechmann's Plasmogen and Dechmann's Tonogen, at intervals varying from a half to two hours.

The treatment, let me repeat, must depend upon the temperament and strength of the patient. The quiet energetic person can endure energetic packs. His body may be completely packed, or at least three quarters, by placing wet and dry sheets around the entire body except the arms, while a woollen blanket is wrapped around the whole body including the arms, or the arms may be left free under the bed clothes. A patient of this type may also be treated with ablutions or put into a half bath at 75 degrees, while cooler water is poured over him. Young and robust patients can endure even cooler baths, which act as a powerful stimulant.

The weaker and more nervous a patient is, the greater caution must be exercised in the use of baths. Such a patient should be given only lukewarm baths, or ablutions at 77 degrees, which may be made to exert a greater stimulus by not drying him. The frequent washing of hands, face and neck, without drying them, is very beneficial to weak patients. Clean, well combed hair also soothes. Slight ablutions of the head, and combing the hair while it is wet, are very refreshing and cooling, especially to women.

What has been said with regard to the treatment of fever may be summarized thus: In the treatment of a strong patient one can rely upon a vigorous procedure. Cold packs may be applied if the fever is very high ; every half hour or hour, or at intervals of an hour and a half to two hours when the fever is not so high. With persons of a weaker constitution, less energetic and more varied treatment is required. Mild ablutions several times a day, with occasional packs on the lower part of the body, or on the calves of the legs. Cool or cold enemas have a quieting influence on the large blood reservoir in the abdomen. Too much water weakens the patient, therefore, only a very little at a time should be given as a drink.

As indicated above, fever is a state of excitement, an internal revolution, which differs so greatly as to cause and in degree, that it cannot be judged or treated according to any fixed rule. The significance of fever depends, of course, upon the temperament and the strength of the various organs of a patient. In other words, our treatment of fever in a specific case must be determined by the power of resistance possessed by the patient.

III.

It is essential that the supply of vital force, but that of the nerves in particular, shall be increased speedily, and for this purpose nothing better can be obtained than Dechmanna Egg Punch. The method of preparing this, and the directions for its use follow :

Take one dozen of absolutely fresh eggs, separate the whites from the yolks very carefully, and beat the yolks into a fine emulsion. In the meantime, take one pound of sugar in a pint of water and boil until a rich syrup is obtained. Then pour the still warm syrup slowly into the egg-yolk emulsion, stirring it continually so that there is a perfect combination of the yolk and syrup. Have your physician prescribe for you a pint of Elixir aromatic, U. S. Pharmacopoeia, and mix this with the emulsion of egg yolk and syrup.

This divine Ambrosia is at once medicine and food. Take a sherry glass full three times a day. It can be made more appetizing and more nourishing by beating the whites of the egg to a froth and serving a little on top of each glass.

In explanation of the great restorative value of Dechmanna Egg Punch, consider these facts: The yolk of a fresh egg contains about one gram of pure lecithin—that is, pure nerve fat—which is absolutely essential to supply the nerves with energy and material for combustion. It also contains organic iron which is indispensible for binding the inhaled oxygen. Moreover, it contains in organic form all of the minerals essential for the upbuilding of new cells in the body. The sugar syrup acts both as a preservative of albumen and as a generator of bodily heat. The etheric oils in the Elixir aromatic are the finest nerve stimulants known to the science of physiological chemistry.

How does it succeed in helping to tone up and restore the depleted Vagus nerve?

When this Ambrosia is digested and assimilated it courses through the lymph channels and lacteal vessels and by the familiar route followed by the chyle enters the heart, where it joins the blood. In the arterial blood it is carried to all parts of the body, including the external glands, and thus aids in energizing the Vagus nerve and all its accessories. Once in circulation, it bursts into the pancreas and other glands, and the intestines, mingles with the secretions of the glands, with the oily salts of the bile, and any impurities (auto-toxins) it finds are driven in the form of excrement and urine out of the system.

This indicates that it acts upon the whole physiological process at one sweep. Thus the bowels and kidneys are assisted in performing their functions properly, and the destructive and poisonous results of catabolism are speedily removed from the body. What course of therapeutic action could be more rational?

Compare this for a moment with the usual method of treating the disease. The result of this method is to tone up the system, to refresh the nerves by supplying material with which to make good the waste incident to disease, and to aid the circulation of the blood. The usual practice, on the other hand, is to prescribe drugs which either whip the famished nerves into activity or else narcotize them. Aspirin, a rank concoction, is a favorite, though it will ruin any digestive tract. Anti-febrine, Anti-pyrine, Codein, Heroin— so the list runs. Not one of them possesses the power to add a single atom to the vital force. On the contrary, every one of them serves but to narcotize, to stifle the spark in the already weakened and overburdened nerves.

In addition to what is said about diet, it should be borne in mind always that a pure atmosphere rich in oxygen is one of the principal remedies demanded in the treatment of diseases of the nerves, lungs and larynx. Those affected with diseases of these organs must avoid drafts and sudden changes in temperature, and should make it an inflexible rule to live in rooms where the temperature is equable.

At this point let me suggest a dietetic scheme for use in the treatment of influenza. It will be noted that the regime includes the use of pack while the patient is awake. This is, of course, to be applied in the manner already described.

The daily regime follows :

For breakfast : A bowl of milk toast with a piece of butter melted on it.
At 10 *a.m.:* A sherry glass of Dech-manna Egg punch with a Graham cracker.
At noon: A bowl of strengthening soup with a piece of buttered toast.*
2 *to* 4 *p. m. :* Abdominal pack.
At 4 *p. m. :* A sherry glass of Dech-manna Egg Punch with a Graham cracker.
At 7 *p.m.:* A cup of custard with a slice of buttered toast.
At 10 *p. m. :* A sherry glass of Dech-manna Egg Punch with a Graham cracker.

After the patient has partaken of food, a piece of extra thick woollen cloth should be warmed and placed over the abdomen for about an hour.

The strengthening soup: Three pounds of fresh beef bones broken into inch pieces by the butcher, and with a pound of brisket added, after a thorough washing in cold water, should be put in enough cold water to cover them and allowed to stew for several hours. Now take soup vegetables, such as parsley, celery, onions, carrots, leeks, turnips, and others ; chop them fine, suspend them in a cloth bag in the broth, and boil for two or three hours. Then take off the stove, strain the broth through a cloth and put in a stone jar. This is a gelatinous stock rich in organic minerals.

For each day, take a third of the stock, add a little water, bits of egg, barley, sago, vermicelli, etc., and finish cooking. Flavor with a little salt. The ingredients added to the daily portion of this soup should be varied so as to avoid having the patient quickly tire of it. Hard toast or zwieback should always be eaten with soup, so as to salivate it properly.

The albumen and marrow of joints is readily transformed into blood gelatine. It requires very little change in the process of digestion to prepare it for absorption by the lymph vessels of the intestines, which suck up the chyle.

In those States where the Elexir aromatic cannot be lawfully prescribed, the Dech-manna Egg Punch may be prepared as follows:

Take one quart of simple syrup and a dozen fresh eggs prepared as already described. Then mix and dissolve the following etheric oils in quantity of lemon extract stated below, and pour the whole slowly into the syrupy emulsion of egg-yolk and simple syrup :

Oil of Orange : 10 drops.

/41

Oil of Coriander : 1 drop.
Oil of Anise : 1 drop.
Lemon Extract : 18 drops.

Put a spoonful of beaten white of egg on top of each glass of Dech-manna Egg Punch, and add a dash of grated nutmeg.

In the therapeautic measures described thus far in this chapter I have endeavored to show how we may check the development of incipient influenza, and how we can avert the dangers attendant upon its development if we are belated in discovering that we are in its grip. It is quite impossible, of course, to discuss every phase of the disease and its treatment in detail within the compass of this booklet.

The question of complications, for instance, is so broad that a discussion of it would take far more space than the booklet contains. It is discussed fully in the second edition of "Dare to be Healthy," a simple compendium of information on biology and physiological chemistry. A copy of this work may be had for the asking.

The author does not practice medicine, does not visit patients. He is a counselor in biology and physiological chemistry. If the physician in charge desires he will consult with him about the application of the principles outlined herein to the treatment of patients suffering from influenza.

IV.

In the light of what has been revealed with regard to the functions of the Vagus nerve and the development of influenza, the bacillus should be forever left inside the covers of learned books on bacteriology. It has been but a poor apology for an explanation of the disease to which human flesh is heir !

The searching light of chemistry reveals to us clearly that the problems in disease are to be solved only by stopping chemical decomposition of the blood, and it shows us how to accomplish this.

I have sought to apply the principals of physiological chemistry to the diagnosis and treatment of influenza. I know that I have not only succeeded in throwing some light upon this darkest of all epidemics, but have explained the underlying cause of it, and my task is finished. Philosophy teaches us that knowledge is like love, a veritable paradox, in that we can only preserve it by giving it away. Such knowledge as I have, I give freely to humanity.

"Primum est humanitas,

Secundum scientia. "

February 1st, 1919.

127 North 59th Street.   Telephone: Ballard 2274.

Seattle, Washington, U. S. A.

Note

* The recipe for making the strengthening soup mentioned in the above dietary appears a little further on. Also a recipe for making Dech-manna Egg Punch in those States where the physician is forbidden to prescribe the Elixir aromatic of the U. S. Pharmacopoeia.

www.ingramcontent.com/pod-product-compliance
Lightning Source LLC
Chambersburg PA
CBHW071436200326
41520CB00014B/3723